The Enlightened Climber

Scaling the Heights with Buddha

Table of Contents

Chapter 1. Introduction

Dive into a unique fusion of the physical and spiritual with our Special Report: "The Enlightened Climber: Scaling the Heights with Buddha." Journey alongside daring adventurers as they harness the wisdom of Buddha, intertwining mindfulness and fortitude to conquer Earth's most formidable peaks. This isn't your typical mountaineering guide; it's a transformative exploration that marries the ascent of challenging landscapes with the transcendental ascent towards enlightenment. You'll be captivated by enthralling narratives, breathtaking photographs, and profound insights - a potent cocktail designed to elevate your spirit and inspire your own quest for enlightenment, no matter what mountains you may face in your life. Get ready to embark on a journey of body, mind, and soul, a delightful adventure with impact beyond the summits. The Enlightened Climber awaits you; don't miss this extraordinary opportunity to climb higher, in more ways than one!

Chapter 2. The Foundations of Buddhist Wisdom

Buddhist wisdom forms the bedrock of the Enlightened Climber's journey: it guides one's relationship with the self and the world, beautifying the harshness of the climb and tempering the sharpness of the wind. This wisdom is grounded in the teachings of Gautama Buddha and the structures of thought that have been carefully built around his teachings, inching humanity towards liberation – nirvana. As climbers, we too seek liberation: from fear, self-doubt, and physical limitation. Through examining the core tenets of Buddhist wisdom – the Four Noble Truths, the Noble Eightfold Path, and the concept of emptiness – we find our climbing experiences imbued with a profound transcendental resonance.

2.1. The Four Noble Truths

Gautama Buddha's first sermon after his enlightenment was the discourse on the Four Noble Truths, a foundational construct of Buddhist philosophy. It provides a succinct diagnosis of the human condition and outlines the path towards liberation.

The first truth, dukkha, often translates as suffering but encapsulates the entire spectrum of unsatisfactory experiences, from mild discomfort to the most excruciating pain. As climbers, we're no strangers to dukkha, from the physical strain during ascents to the mental anxiety of navigating treacherous terrains.

The second truth, samudaya, identifies the root cause of suffering - attachment and desire, often compounded by ignorance of their effects. Our climbing endeavors can be plagued by attachment to outcomes: the allure of the summit, the fear of failure, or egoistic competition.

The third truth, nirodha, holds the promise of cessation of suffering. This is the state of Nirvana – a liberation from all attachments and therefore from all forms of suffering.

The fourth truth, mārga, provides a practical roadmap to reach Nirvana – through the Noble Eightfold Path, which we delve into next.

2.2. The Noble Eightfold Path

The climber's route to spiritual enlightenment through Buddhist wisdom involves a rigorous climb along the Noble Eightfold Path, a comprehensive guidance system for moral, mental, and intellectual development.

Right view, the first step, is the comprehension of the Four Noble Truths. It underlines the necessity of understanding our experiences on the mountain as part of the broader existential landscape.

Right intention, the second step, is the commitment to ethical and mental self-improvement. For climbers, this encapsulates intentions of goodwill, renunciation, and harmlessness, essential in our exchanges with nature and fellow climbers.

Ethical conduct is addressed in the next three steps: right speech, right action, and right livelihood. Climbers manifest these in their actions, conversations, and even in their role in the climbing community.

Right effort, the sixth step, concerns self mastery. Climbers experience this through training, the disciplined mind on the route, and the resolve to move forward despite adversity.

Right mindfulness, the seventh step, involves clear awareness of one's body, feelings, mind, and phenomena. The necessity of mindfulness in climbing can't be overstated; every hold, every step, and every breath requires acute awareness.

Finally, right concentration, or meditation, necessitates focusing the mind single-pointedly on a serene and wholesome object for clarity and tranquillity.

Through these eight steps, climbers can cultivate an inner sanctuary of peace even when pitted against the harshest natural forces.

2.3. The Concept of Emptiness

In Buddhist philosophy, emptiness, or Sunyata, signifies the interdependence of all phenomena and the absence of any singular, inherent essence. This underlines the impermanence of all things; the constantly changing bodily states while climbing, the transitory nature of the mountain, even the fleeting triumph at the summit.

Grasping emptiness allows us to disconnect from our egocentric perspectives. It frees us from the bindings of the self, releasing us into the boundless panorama of existence. This helps us understand and appreciate the magnificent interplay between us, as climbers, and the mountains, resulting in a genuine connectedness that elevates the climbing experience.

In the following chapters, we will delve into the practical applications of these concepts to our mountaineering journeys. While the path may be steep and strenuous, remember, it is through these arduous climbs that we internalize the profound wisdom of Buddha, scale the heights of our existence, and stride towards spiritual liberation. Let every step turn the wheel of Dharma, let every breath kindle the flame of enlightenment.

Chapter 3. Training the Mind: Meditation Techniques for the Adventurous Climber

Mountaineering isn't merely a physical challenge; it's a sophisticated dance of the mind and spirit. Sharp, alert minds safeguard the body against the perils of altitude, cold, and fatigue. The wisdom of Buddha offers central tenets to refine such mental fortitude and direct your journey. However, the process requires practice.

Embedding practice in your climbing preparation is like training a muscle. Just as you wouldn't attempt Everest without physical preparedness, so too must the mind be conditioned for the singular demands of elevated climes. Here, we present some integral methods rooted in Buddhist philosophy to augment your mountaineering journey.

3.1. Mindfulness: A Basecamp for the Mind

The roots of mindfulness lie in Buddhism where it has been recognized as a crucial element of the path to enlightenment. It involves non-judgmental, active attention to the present moment, thus anchoring the mind and enabling clarity and calm. How can this serve trekkers about to embark on a daunting expedition?

Pre-climb, mindfulness engenders a keen awareness of your body's signals, promoting acute discernment of readiness or potential issues before they spiral. On the mountain, it keeps the mind firmly rooted in the present, averting harmful distractions and minimizing stress. The present is all there is on the mountain, and mindfulness markedly aids in aligning your mental energies with this reality.

To incorporate mindfulness practice, follow these guidelines:

1. Tune into your breath: Settle comfortably, closing your eyes, drawing attention to the breath. Observe the rise and fall of your chest, the air whipping past your nostrils. If your mind drifts, gently draw it back.

2. Body scanning: Start from your toes, working up. Notice sensations – tingling, pressure, warmth. Recognize these feelings without attachment or judgement.

3. Mindful eating: As you eat, focus on each bite – the flavor, texture, and the sensation of swallowing.

4. Attentive walking: As you train, focus on your step – the ground beneath the foot, shift in your muscles, rhythm of your stride.

3.2. Equanimity: Sailing Through the Storms

Equanimity, or the art of mental balance, is another Buddhist principle you can adopt. Life throws adversity at us. So do mountains. The ability to maintain composure during tumultuous times and not get carried away with success can be lifesaving while climbing.

Practicing mental composure starts in day-to-day life. Detach from emotional reactions-joy, anger, worry, or anticipation. Accept that events happen. You can't control them but can control your reactions. To strengthen this skill, try a basic meditation: relax, breathe, and focus the mind. Acknowledge thoughts, feelings, without reaction nor suppression. Imagine them as clouds passing by in your mental sky. Return to focusing on the breath.

3.3. The Mantras: The Mental Carabiners

Mantras, integral to Buddhism, denote a phrase or sound repeated to aid concentration. For climbers, it acts as mental carabiners that lock their minds to the climb, preventing hazardous mental meandering.

Repetition of a mantra ties you to the present, offering a mechanism analogous to an anchor in a tumultuous sea. Additionally, mantra repetition reinforces meaningful concepts, feeding your motivation and drive. Consider phrases that resonate with you personally - "Fear is temporary, summits are eternal," or simple sounds, like - "Om."

3.4. Compassion and Loving-Kindness: The Balm for Suffering

Bringing compassion to the fore in your climbing journey serves dual fronts. First, it intimately ties you to your fellow climbers, fostering interdependence, critical to any team-based alpine endeavor. Second, it reframes the internal dialogue - you're more patient with yourself, accepting your unique pace and ability, mitigating stress and resentment.

Loving-kindness meditation – wishing happiness, health, safety, and ease to others and yourself – can further augment compassion:

1. Breath calmly and visualize someone you care deeply about. Wish them happiness, health, and peace.

2. Repeat this process for yourself, someone neutral to you, someone you struggle with, and finally all sentient beings.

3.5. Emptiness: Let Go, Climb High

Buddhism teaches us about 'Shunyata' or emptiness. It encapsulates the concept of letting go, untying ourselves from rigid views or attachments. This enables greater flexibility and resilience. A climber clinging to fixed expectations of weather or physical conditions may be less prepared for unexpected changes or setbacks.

Emptiness meditation involves observing thoughts and perceptions, contemplating their transient, unfixed nature. This aids in developing a flexible mindset, ready for whatever the mountain might offer.

Buddhist techniques aren't mere band-aid solutions but tools of transformation. They can redefine the essence of your climb, turning it from a physical feat to a remarkable spiritual journey, enabling you to touch not just the highest peaks of the Earth but also the zeniths of your inner self. Practicing these techniques can unlock the enlightened climber within you. Now start training your mind, as you would your body.

Chapter 4. Mindful Mountaineering: Applying Awareness on the Ascent

It is in the nature of Himalayan sages and alpinists alike that they discover within themselves a kind of interior terrain, which provides the stamina to resist the pull of defeat, the resilience to endure privation, and the audacity to face down fear. At the intersection of these seemingly disparate paths lays Mindful Mountaineering: a technique that catapults climbers past physical limitations and into a consideration of climbing as a spiritual undertaking.

4.1. Understanding Mindful Mountaineering

In essence, mindful mountaineering refers to a conscious approach to scaling mountains that concentrates on the present moment, excluding any other distractions. Once you've grasped the concept, the practice is relatively straightforward. By focusing on your immediate surrounds - the rock beneath your fingertips, the ground under your boots, the wind against your skin - you learn to drown out superfluous thoughts and give your all to the task at hand.

Pulling these two strands together, mindfulness and mountaineering, requires a subtle shift in perspective. It's about learning to see mountaineering not just as a physical challenge, but a spiritual journey that can lead towards greater self-awareness and clarity.

4.2. The Importance of Being Present

The value of staying present when climbing can't be overstated. Every foothold and handhold matter, and if you're not fully invested in the moment, you can easily misjudge a grip or step. This awareness extends beyond the physical, providing space to calmly process fear, excitement or fatigue, without allowing these emotions to consume or derail us.

Staying present requires learning to put aside thoughts of the summit or the route ahead, and instead focus on the now. This is easier said than done; it requires diligence, practice, and a certain amount of mental discipline.

Moreover, being in the present moment can facilitate a deep communion with nature. It sharpens your senses to the rustling leaves, the whispering wind, the distant chirping of a hillside bird, or the quiet trickle of a near-frozen stream – stimuli that you might overlook when lost in ego-driven goal pursuit.

4.3. Harnessing Breath

One of the most effective ways to practice mindfulness while climbing is to focus on breath. Breathing controls our stress levels and aids recovery after a strenuous stretch. When we pay attention to our breath, we achieve two things: we slow our heart rate, which helps to steady us, and we remind ourselves of the embodiment and the impermanence of our existence, promoting our connection to the world around us.

When you are climbing, notice the rise and fall of your breath. Feel the cool intake of oxygen, hold onto it for a second, and then let it rush out. With each inhale, we fill our bodies with needed oxygen, and with each exhale, we release tension.

4.4. Practicing Gratitude

Gratitude, while often overlooked, can significantly improve our climbing experience. Before you begin your climb, take a few minutes to stand at the base of the peak and express silent gratitude. Be thankful for your health that allows you to climb, the beauty of nature around you, the opportunity to challenge yourself, and the periods of tranquility you will find on your ascent.

4.5. Acceptance and Letting Go

Mindful mountaineering isn't just about being aware of the present—it's also about accepting what comes and letting go of what we can't control. Despite hours spent meticulously prepping for the climb, there will be variables beyond your control. This could be a sudden shift in the weather or equipment malfunction. In these moments, acceptance is crucial. You cannot change the situation but can change how you react to it.

4.6. Deep Listening to Your Body

As climbers, we often push our bodies beyond measurable limits. We nurture the capacity to endure physical discomfort, because we understand that climbing demands it. But mindful mountaineering redirects us away from this grim control over our bodies, and instead advocates deep, empathetic listening. Are we close to an injury? Are we genuinely thirsty, or do we just crave the comfort of a water break? By tuning in, we can better care for our bodies, ensuring they can support us through to the summit, and beyond.

Mindful mountaineering isn't a checklist or a set technique. It's an approach, a mindset. Embrace it not to become a better climber, but to enrich your climbing experience. As you ascend, remember that the peak isn't all there is. The slope is the journey, and every stone, every cloud, every gust of wind has stories to tell you about the world and about yourself. Be there, fully and completely, on your climbs. For in the journey and not the summit, lies the true joy of mountaineering.

Chapter 5. Facing The Elements: Courage and Compassion in the Face of Adversity

Our journey begins in the predawn darkness, high on the flank of Mount Everest, where the hostile environs challenge even the hardiest of adventurers. The air, thin to the edge of nonexistence, struggles to offer up the fleeting molecules of oxygen climbers desperately need. The lofty peak remains shrouded in the obscurity of the waning night, its devastatingly magnificent glaciers, a relentlessly frozen riverscape illuminated by the waxing crescent moon.

5.1. The Beauty and Brutality of Everest

This, the world's highest peak, is brutally indifferent. Given life by the towering grandeur of the Himalayas, Everest has seen countless climbers embrace its flanks over the decades, drawn to its proverbial summit experience. Yet it stands, both beautiful and brutal, never yielding before the frail courage of the climbers, exacting a toll for every inch conceded. Mountaineers have always been on a quest to conquer it, but this journey explores how Buddhist teachings infuse the ascent with spiritual significance, lending wisdom to courage, and compassion to strength.

For a Buddhist climber, Everest is not just a physical landmark to be conquered. It is a metaphor for the human struggle against adversity, for the bravery required in the face of fear, for the compassion necessary when facing the harsh realities of life. Here, we find not only courage and compassion but the quintessential essence of Buddhism itself.

5.2. Buddhism: A Life Philosophy

The pillars of Buddhism, the Four Noble Truths, provide a profound roadmap to enlightenment. It addresses the suffering that is an inescapable part of life, illustrates the causes of this suffering, and offers a liberating path, the Eightfold Path. The ultimate goal is to extinguish the flames of desire, ignorance, and hatred, breaking the chains of karma and rebirth, achieving a state beyond suffering: Nirvana. Buddhism, then, is more than just a religion, it is a philosophy of life, a guide through the tumultuous seas of existence.

Applying this to mountaineering, we, the climbers, are on a journey that perfectly illustrates these teachings. Each step is a movement towards understanding, acceptance, and liberation. In conquering Everest, climbers are not just defeating a formidable physical challenge but are also navigating the harsh terrains of their minds, their fears, their prejudices, and their ignorances.

5.3. Courage under the Zen Shadow

Many may question: can courage exist under the serene gaze of Buddhism? Does the conquering spirit have a place within the Buddhist philosophy of accepting, letting go, and ultimate detachment?

Buddhism does not view courage as brashness or bravado. Instead, courage is perceived from a standpoint of wisdom and compassion. This form of courage emphasizes moving forward despite fear, understanding the ephemeral nature of life and death, and caring deeply and selflessly for all living beings, including oneself. The courage of a climber entwined with the Buddha's teachings, remains rooted in mindfulness and a wholesome understanding of the mountain they undertake to conquer.

5.4. Compassion: The Heart of the Climb

Compassion, synonymous with Buddhism, extends beyond mere sympathy. It is the active desire to alleviate the suffering of ourselves and others. For a climber nurturing the seed of compassion within, each step up the mountain resonates with this intent. Climbers not only reach out to fellow mountaineers but also establish a connection with the mountain itself, seeing it as a living, breathing entity deserving respect and care.

5.5. Understanding Impermanence

Another fundamental aspect to discourse, as we ascend in this physical and spiritual journey, is the Buddhist concept of impermanence. No summit once reached stays conquered forever, like no sorrow or joy remains unchanging. A climber with a Buddhist mindset understands this deeply. He knows the summit remains where it is, just as the valley remains where it is. It's the climber alone who moves through this transient existence. This transiency may be unsettling for some, but through Buddhist teachings, it becomes a source of liberation, a means of breaking free from the cycles of suffering.

Now, as our enlightened climbers embrace Everest in the predawn light, understanding its beauty, accepting its cruelty, and deeply feeling the transient nature of all existence, they breathe life into the symbiotic fusion of mind, body, and spirit. Challenge and serenity, physicality and spirituality, effort and acceptance, they become the counterpoints of a complex melody that echoes the teachings of Buddha against the vastness of the open skies and the timelessness of the mountains. This journey is not just about conquering the peak of

Everest, it's about experiencing the journey and understanding the true nature of life and existence, the very essence of Buddhism.

Stay with us as we further delve into the intertwined paths of spirituality and physical might in the next chapter. As we continue to scale the heights with Buddha, remember that the summit isn't necessarily the destination; it's the journey and the enlightenment that follows it that truly matters.

Chapter 6. Beyond Fear: The Buddhist Approach to Overcoming Climbing Challenges

As any climber knows, the physical and technical aspects of mountaineering are only half of the battle. The other half is mental — grappling with the fear and anxiety that can halt climbers in their tracks, leading to doubt and, potentially, danger. In this chapter, we will explore the Buddhist perspective on fear and the techniques that can help us confront and overcome it, transforming it from a hindrance to a tool for deeper understanding and personal growth.

6.1. The Nature of Fear

Understanding fear from a Buddhist perspective requires a shift in thought: fear is not an adversary but a fundamental aspect of our human condition. Fear is a distinct form of suffering or "Dukkha," a central Buddhist concept, denoting the existential unsatisfactoriness and discontent arising from the impermanent and imperfect nature of worldly life.

The Buddha identified two types of fear: 'healthy' fear, which is a rational response to a direct and immediate threat, and 'unhealthy' fear, which springs from our imagination and speculation about the future. Much of the fear experienced in mountain climbing falls into the latter category. The incessant "what-ifs" can chip away at your confidence, creating an invisible but insurmountable wall between you and your goal.

6.2. Perceiving Fear through the Four Noble Truths

To process fear through the lens of Buddhism, we can utilize the Four Noble Truths. These truths are the Buddha's basic teachings, laying out the problem of suffering, its causes, its cessation, and the path to its cessation.

First, the truth of suffering or Dukkha includes fear. To deny it, to suppress it, or to run from it merely perpetuates the cycle of suffering. Accepting fear as an integral part of your journey is the first step toward overcoming it.

Second, the truth of the cause of Dukkha: in the context of fear, you can understand this as attachment to particular outcomes or aversion to potential dangers. When you're hanging onto a sheer cliff face, fear can bloom from your attachment to reaching the summit, or your revulsion toward the drop beneath you.

Third, the truth of the cessation of suffering: just as fear arises, it can also cease. This is the promise that gives us hope and the goal we work towards.

Finally, the truth of the path leading to cessation of Dukkha: This leads us to the Eightfold Path, a practical guide to liberating oneself from suffering.

6.3. Following the Eightfold Path

The Eightfold Path is the practice that transforms understanding into lived experience. Implementing them in our climbing practice might look as follows:

- Right Understanding: Recognize that your fear is a form of suffering nand comes from your attachments and aversions.

- Right Thought: Maintain a mindset of open curiosity toward your fear, rather than hostility or denial.

- Right Speech: Articulate your fears honestly, without exaggeration or minimization.

- Right Action: Consciously regulate your actions, not letting them be controlled by fear.

- Right Livelihood: Choose ascents that align with your skills, strengths, and values – not solely for pride or recognition.

- Right Effort: Endeavor to acknowledge and dissolve fear whenever it arises.

- Right Mindfulness: Stay present with fear, not fleeing into fantasies of past or future.

- Right Concentration: Focus continuously on the present moment, the presence of fear, and the overcoming of fear.

6.4. Incorporating Mindfulness Into Your Climb

Mindfulness is the heart of the Buddha's teachings and is underpinned by the concepts of awareness and attention. Bringing mindfulness into your climb involves focusing on the present, not ruminating on past failures, or anxiously anticipating future obstacles.

Mindful climber learns to climb 'in the moment,' which not only improves focus, accuracy, and efficiency but also gradually dispels fear. Mindful breathing, for example, can not only stabilize erratic heartbeats but can also ease the mind. By focusing attention on breath – the inhale and exhale – you anchor yourself in the present, diffusing the worry about future unknowns.

6.5. Applying Metta (Loving-Kindness) To Self And Others

In the face of fear, metta - or loving-kindness - can be a compelling antidote. It starts with extending kindness and understanding towards ourselves in our fear. From this place of self-compassion, we can extend that same unconditional care towards our climbing partners, creating a supportive environment conducive to progress and safety.

Remember, fear doesn't make you weak – it makes you human. By engaging with Buddhist philosophy and practices, you can reshape your relationship with fear, learning to work with it and through it. The Enlightened Climber knows that the mountains we fear are often the ones in our minds – making the journey not just one of physical elevation, but of personal evolution, wisdom, and enlightenment.

Chapter 7. The Summit Within: Achieving Inner Peaks Through Mindfulness

It may seem logical to consider the physical conquest of a mountain peak the ultimate achievement. Yet, in the world of the Enlightened Climber, summiting the mountainous exterior is just the precursor to another, more significant summit within. This interior journey, which carries us across the terrains of self-awareness and into the universe of the present moment, is often more formidable than any landscape nature can present.

7.1. Trekking Through Mindfulness: A Basic Primer

Mindfulness, in simplest terms, is a conscious, non-judgmental awareness of the present moment. It is the cultivation of an acute attention to our experiences - our thoughts, feelings, and sensory data - without trying to alter or resist them. In the context of mountaineering, it means fully immersing oneself in the act of climbing, letting the worries of the future or the regrets of the past fade into insignificance.

Let's explore this concept further using the primary tools of mindfulness: the breath and the body.

7.2. Harnessing the Breath: Your Steadiest Rope

The breath is a climber's greatest ally. It doesn't merely keep us alive; it can also become a lifeline to the elusive present moment. While climbing, pay attention to every inhalation and exhalation. Feel your lungs expand and contract, your chest rise and fall. Notice the cycle, the rhythm, and the life-sustaining dance of respiration.

A focus on the breath performs two vital tasks for a climber. Firstly, it anchors you to the present moment, pulling your mind away from unnecessary anxieties about the climb's outcome or the echoes of past failures. Secondly, it aids in regulating your metabolism, helping you conserve energy and maintain the necessary endurance for your physical journey.

7.3. Bodily Awareness: Ascending with every Step

Take a moment, wherever you are on your trek, to be silent and invite your attention to every detail of your body. Noticing bodily sensations enhances your connection with the terrain you're in. It develops a fundamental recognition of the balance between your body and the rocky environment, awakening a profound reverence for both.

Feel the frigid winds slapping against your face or an unwelcome fatigue pulsating in your calves. Don't judge or resist these sensations; instead, observe them with a calm curiosity, an explorer's dedication. This observational stance can deliver surprising jolts of energy that can propel you at moments when the climb feels unbearable.

Your body is the vehicle to your external and internal summits. By fostering bodily awareness, you fortify this vehicle, making it ready for the challenges that lie ahead.

7.4. The Mind-Mountain Symbiosis: Interchange of Lessons

The mountain, though silent, is a wise teacher. Steep slopes teach resilience, paralyzing cold urges adaptability, and unpredictable turns awaken alertness. By being mindful and present in your ascent, you expose yourself to these vital lessons, allowing them to permeate your consciousness.

On the other hand, the mind, in its tranquility, can influence your perception of the mountain. When the mind is calm and present, even the daunting rocky behemoth turns into a field of learning, adventure, and self-discovery. In this way, a symbiosis forms between your mind and the mountain - an orchestration of wisdom and action.

7.5. Summiting Your Inner Peaks: Liberating Possibilities

Mindful mountaineering is not about conquering but about understanding. By understanding the mountain, you gain wisdom, and by understanding yourself, you attain freedom. Concepts such as fear, failure, and success find new meaning on this journey. The rigors of the physical climb provide a stage on which these constructs unveil their falseness and transient nature.

The inner summit reveals itself when you dismantle these constructs. And once at this pinnacle, you find yourself radically restructured. The sense of self extends beyond your ego. You find yourself inextricably connected to the mountain, the wind, the earth, and every living being on this planet. It is this interconnectedness that brings forth an unparalleled sense of liberation.

Indeed, mindfulness doesn't make the climb easy; it makes it transformative. As you scale each physical and emotional peak with unwavering awareness, you approach not just the mountain's summit, but also the zenith of your potential. You commune not only with nature's grandeur but also your astounding innate capacities.

7.6. The Enlightened Climber: A Catalyst for Change

As climbers, our potentiality for change is limitless. Our every encounter with the ascent can be a catalyst for transformation. By intertwining the physical voyage with an internal pilgrimage, we become more than mere mountaineers. We morph into entities of change - embodiments of resilience, wisdom, and infinite possibility, transcending the average human experience.

The Enlightened Climber, armed with an adventurous spirit and unwavering mindfulness, ceaselessly quests towards newer dimensions, stretching the limits of the possible. He goes beyond exploring new landscapes to unearthing latent aspects of the self. He is, thus, not just a climber of mountains but a conqueror of his interior frontiers, a true pioneer who blazes trails into uncharted territories of human potential.

In this sense, scaling a mountain becomes a metaphor for life. It rescues us from the monotony of our routines and thrusts us into a thrilling ballet of uncertainty and discovery. It pushes us to explore not just nature's majesty but our existence's poignant beauty as well.

At its core, mindful mountaineering is an evolving dialogue between the self and the universe. It nurtures resilience, awareness, and an unquenchable spirit of exploration. Through this marvelous fusion of physical effort and spiritual insight, we all can become Enlightened Climbers, individuals capable of scaling any mountain - whether made of rock or thought - and standing triumphant at those beautiful, enlightened peaks within.

Chapter 8. Climbing Karma: Treading Lightly on The Mountains

In the high-altitude environment, progress is often measured in inches, both literal and figurative. The peaks we conquer manifest the outward expression of internal triumph, a hard won victory over not just the elements, but also over our own fears, doubts, and limitations. However, in the act of conquering, we must remember our duties and responsibilities towards these majestic behemoths of nature. In this light, 'Climbing Karma: Treading Lightly on The Mountains' signifies an enlightened approach to mountaineering, where every climb is not an act of dominance, but a humble quest for personal growth and spiritual enlightenment.

8.1. Start Where You Stand

Buddha pointedly remarked, "There is no path to happiness: happiness is the path." In the context of climbing, the lesson is clear. The joy is not in reaching the summit, but in every step taken towards it. How we approach our climbing endeavors can profoundly shape not only the journey itself but also our perception of the world.

Before scaling a mountain, examine your motivations. Are you hoping to conquer the peak, to dominate and assert your superiority over it? Do you seek the thrill of risk, or the silence of solitude? Or are you there to witness the sublime beauty? A coherent philosophy of approach becomes an inner compass, guiding us to act respectably and consciously throughout the journey, thereby creating positive 'climbing karma'.

Respect should extend to the communities inhabiting these regions.

For them, the mountains may embody homes, identities, or even religious deities. Engage with them, comprehend their customs, traditions, and beliefs, and incorporate these lessons into your climbing philosophy. Such an approach transforms mountaineering from a mere sport into a nuanced cultural and spiritual experience.

8.2. On The Intrinsic Value of Mountains

According to Buddhist teachings, all beings have Buddha-nature, an inherently enlightened essence. Now, consider the mountain. It does not seek attention or beg for validation; it merely exists. It stands both formidable and serene, a testament to natural beauty and strength.

To view mountains as mere climbing destinations is to belittle their essence. Instead, appreciate their intrinsic value. This perspective fosters reverence and respect towards the environment. It promotes responsible behavior, such as practicing 'Leave No Trace' principles, minimizing environmental degradation. By aiming to leave the mountains as we found them, we ensure their preservation for future generations.

8.3. Resilience: More than Physical Strength

The essential character of a climber is no different from that of a mountain. Both must withstand the harshest conditions. However, resilience is a trait measured not just in physical endurance, but also in mental and spiritual strength.

In the face of adversity, it's natural to question your abilities, to entertain doubts about the journey. The key, as Buddha instructed, is to accept these thoughts, not suppress them. Recognizing uncertainties allows us to treat them as impermanent phenomena — rising and fading, but never defining our capabilities or planning.

Resilience also entails respecting our limits. Refusing to risk life and limb in pursuit of victory is not a sign of weakness, but wisdom. Withdrawal can be the bravest choice, embodying the Buddhist principle of Ahimsa—non-violence—not only towards others, but towards ourselves as well.

8.4. The Passage of Time: A Climb is a Journey

There's a Buddhist saying: "Do not dwell in the past, do not dream of the future, concentrate the mind on the present moment." Every climb is a journey in time, the path from the base to the summit measuring not just distance, but experiences.

Realizing this allows us to relax into the rhythm of mountain climbing. The journey is not a race to the finish; it is an opportunity to embrace each riveting moment's beauty, challenge, and change. This mindfulness helps us nurture a stronger relationship with nature, ourselves, and our fellow climbers, allowing us to tread lightly on the mountain, leaving no trace but a profound impact on the soul.

8.5. Balance: The Dance Between Effort and Surrender

Striking the right balance between effort and surrender is a key Buddhist teaching that translates seamlessly to mountaineering. Climbers must exert effort to propel themselves upward, but they also need to surrender—accept the realities of the terrain, the weather, and their limitations.

This form of surrender differs from giving up. It is more akin to adaptive resilience—a recognition and acceptance of the reality that allows one to strategize effectively. It signifies wisdom, the ability to understand when to push forward and when to pull back, creating a harmonious dance between action and acceptance.

In the end, the path of the enlightened climber is not marred by dominance, destruction, or disregard. It is an empathetic path, woven with the threads of reverence, respect, and responsibility. It is a transformative journey that challenges us to climb higher, both in altitude and consciousness—the true essence of 'Climbing Karma'.

Chapter 9. Finding Zen at High Altitude: Serenity Amidst the Summits

The mingling of frigid gusts and oxygen-thin air is an arduous trial to the unprepared - a reality known all too well to the high-altitude mountaineer. Yet amidst the looming, snow-blanketed crags, a profound serenity unveils itself, breaking through the physical challenges posed by these colossal geologic marvels. This is the realm where the Enlightened Climber uncovers Zen, on the turbulent precipices and serene plateaus that both test and defy human resilience.

9.1. Embracing the Physical

Zen is often associated with tranquility and peace, seemingly paradoxical to the strenuous ascent up rocky terrain and punishing weather conditions. However, it is precisely in the crux of these adversities that one is afforded the opportunity to cultivate Zen. The physical challenges encountered by climbers are not impediments to attaining Zen but are rather, the very medium for achieving it.

Climbing equates to a deeply personal journey, soliciting from climbers immense physical efforts often paired with discomfort and pain. Yet, leveraging the teachings of Buddha, one can learn to overcome suffering by accepting our physical discomfort, regardless of the dangers—and discomfort—associated with high altitude expeditions.

9.2. Breathing: The Anchor of Present Moment

Buddhist teachings place great emphasis on the act of breathing. Just as it is essential to maintain life, it is a pivotal tool in the pursuit of Zen. At high altitudes, where breath turns sacred, endeavouring to be in synchrony with one's breath is a transformative experience. Each inhale and exhale becomes more precious and tangible, catapulting the importance of one's breathing pattern into clear focus.

In the rarified atmosphere at high altitudes, breath transforms into an ever-present metronome, dictating the rhythm of one's ascend. Given its crucial importance under such circumstances, it only underlines the centrality of breath in the present moment. By focusing on breath control, climbers not only manage the scarcity of oxygen, but also cultivate mindfulness. Each drawn breath becomes a meditative practice, endowing climbers with tranquility amidst the harshness of the mountains.

9.3. Tranquility in Turbulence: The Stoic Resilience

Life in the mountains is far from constant. One moment, the quiet serenity under a starlit night; the next, an incoming storm ready to wreak havoc. The mountains demonstrate to us the impermanence inherent in our existence, a core teaching of Buddha - the doctrine of 'anicca'.

Surviving in such conditions demands a level of stoic resilience, a tranquility in turbulence. Ascending while under duress of an impending storm, climbers learn to silence the chaos of the external environment to retain inner calm. This ability to stay mentally unfazed, even with the onslaught of natural elements, mirrors the Zen philosophy of attaining peace amidst the whirlwind of life's adversities.

9.4. Solitude: A Portal to Inner Reflection

Mountaineering is often a solitary endeavor. The solitude, often viewed negatively in more cosmopolitan contexts, becomes a powerful ally at high altitudes. A solitary trek in the mountains provides a compelling platform for introspection and self-discovery, vital for progressing on the path of enlightenment.

Achieving Zen entails gaining profound insights about oneself; the solitude on the mountaintop becomes a conduit for such reflections. Buddhists seek solitary retreats for in-depth meditation—a practice mountain climbers inadvertently adopt. The quietude and isolation, allowing them to reflect upon their lives, strengths, limitations, fears, and aspirations. It is during these solitary moments that they often encounter profound realizations, experiencing enlightenment amidst the icy peaks.

9.5. Nature: The Impeccable Teacher

In Buddhism, wisdom is understanding the true nature of reality. Mountains, being an integral part of nature, stand as extraordinary teachers. They communicate the reality that everything in this universe is interconnected. Mountaineers live in a symbiotic relationship with the mountain – they prepare, respect, read, and respond to the mountain while navigating its terrain.

The true essence of nature and how it connects to us becomes a powerful teacher in our pursuits to finding Zen. Sensing the subtle shifts in weather patterns, listening to the rumbling of avalanches, and observing the ethereal, mountains assist climbers in their understanding of life. Climbers' respect for mountains deepens as a result of these experiences, fostering a profound sense of awe and appreciation that constitutes part of their enlightening journey.

In concluding, climbing mountains is not merely about reaching the summit but a meditative journey to discover Zen at high altitudes. Each step in this challenging voyage demands resilience, mindfulness, tranquility, introspection, and respect for nature—all aspects intrinsic to Zen and enlightenment. By persevering through perilous terrains and extremities of weather, climbers indeed build toughness. Still, more importantly, they embark on a transformative journey that transcends the physical world, leading them towards the path of spiritual enlightenment.

Chapter 10. The Quiet Strength: Harnessing Silence in Alpine Endeavours

In the grueling escapades of mountain climbing, silence can be a fearsome companion, but if embraced correctly, it becomes an irreplaceable ally. The enormous, imposing peaks, the hardened granulated trails, the biting wind tearing at your layers, all disjointedly come together to paint the milieu of alpine hiking. And cutting across this cacophonous chronicling often comes the eerie silence, accentuating the solitude and laying bare the raw magnitude of the challenges that climbers confront.

10.1. The Paradox of Silence

The deliberate pursuit of silence in mountaineering is paradoxical. Every audacious adventurer stepping onto the hem of this formidable theatre knows the strenuous, physically taxing battles in wait — the relentless grind of hiking, choosing safe paths, setting up camps, battling the brutal weather, and preserving health. A constant dialogue ensues during the climb, boasting of triumphs and shattered vulnerabilities equally.

Yet amidst all the physical exertion and mental gymnastics, the pursuit of silence becomes paramount. For when the tumult in our minds quiets down, the whispers of the mountains become audible; their timeless wisdom navigates us, not only through arduous ascents but our existential worries and soul-searching endeavors.

10.2. Embracing Silence: Lessons from the Buddha

Silence is pervasive in Buddhist teachings and practices. The Buddha, known as the "silent sage," whose teachings provide the bedrock of mindfulness, embraced silence wholly. His quietude was not the disquieting, eerie silence but a peaceful, compassionate one, embodying the essence of enlightenment. The Buddha's teachings guide that silence should not be viewed as an alien presence, but a gateway to mindfulness, bringing us in sync with our existence and the universe.

"How do I embrace silence in mountain climbing?" you might ask. Here lies the beauty of this fusion. It begins with understanding that silence is not an absence but a state of being. It is the rare moments, rising above the jagged terrains and crystal blue glaciers, where one finds peace within the swirling storm of thoughts, encouraging reflection and introspection.

10.3. Harnessing the Power of Silence

There's no dearth of silence on a mountaineering expedition, especially when you're making your solitary path amidst towering peaks. It's the art of utilizing that prevailed silence; the transformative silence that becomes a repository of strength and wisdom.

Firstly, observe the silence. Instead of plugging your ears with music or engrossing in idle chatter, become one with the surrounding quietude. Open your senses to the unperturbed peace, the rustle of the wind, the crunching echo of your boots against the snow, the distant thunderous rumble of a cracking glacier, the rhythmic symphony of your heartbeat and breath.

Secondly, silence is not a void to be filled; rather, it nurtures inner peace. It strengthens the interplay of intuition and improvisation—a lifeline on any climb. The Buddha taught that the more profound the silence, the more luminous the consciousness. Silent moments provide clarity and purge mental fog, instigating sound decisions.

Thirdly, loving silence does not equate to eliminating communication; understanding that dialogue stems from a place of necessity during climbs is crucial. Keeping communications to the essential practice enables the amplification of silence's benefits during climbs.

10.4. Basking in the Quietude: Silence in Solitude

Being alone with one's thoughts, especially in the stark expansiveness of alpine terrains, can become daunting. This eerie solitude, however, is a grace in disguise. It is your tryst with your inner self, the whispers of your soul that get lost in the everyday din.

This solitude offers the perfect opportunity to practice mindful meditation. Rooted in the teachings of the Buddha, mindfulness is the full awareness of the present moment. Becoming aware of your every breath, of the biting cold or the warm sun rays, and even the fatigue creeping into your muscles—the silent observation and acceptance of all sensations, thoughts, and emotions.

Practicing mindfulness in solitude allows climbers to not only master their physical and emotional responses but also foster compassion: towards oneself, towards climbing partners, and towards the mountain. This intense interplay of physical exertion and mental calm paves the path towards enlightenment, making the journey as enriching as summiting the peak itself.

In conclusion, the Buddha's teachings resonate in the silence surrounded by the mightiest peaks, fostering enlightenment beyond conventional wisdom. So harness the power of silence, grow through solitude, and utilize both as stepping stones toward becoming an Enlightened Climber. Through the journey, you will conquer not just towering mountains, but the insurmountable peaks within yourself as well.

Chapter 11. Descending with Dharma: Reflections on a Climbing Journey

The adrenaline rush of standing atop the world's most treacherous peaks is an experience that very few brave hearts can claim to have. Yet, a climber's journey is not merely measured by the victory of the ascent but in the grace of the descent.

11.1. Disconnect to Connect

In an age dominated by technology and constant stimulus, the descent can offer a rare opportunity to disconnect and immerse oneself in the beauty and stillness of nature. As I slowly but surely made my way down, I welcomed the silence. This silence wasn't an absence of sound—it was the absence of noise.

The crunch of my boots against the snow-covered rocks, the distant calls of mountain birds, the soothing whisper of the gentle wind brushing against my cheeks – in the presence of such unfettered rawness, I was able to appreciate the symphony of nature. Alongside this orchestra of organic harmony, the chatter of our mundane worries and anxieties seemed utterly insignificant, as did the pursuits that often preoccupied our daily existence.

Buddha also spoke of this sense of detachment, where he encouraged his disciples to separate from the noise of the world and gravitate towards silence. By unplugging from what we know, focusing on the present moment, we can finally begin to witness the breathtaking expanse of what we do not know.

11.2. Material Simplicity and Spiritual Profundity

Descending the peak did not just entail a lowering of altitude, but it also engendered a profound lowering of oneself. Stripped of my high-tech gear, trading it for simple, warm layers, I began to appreciate the doctrine of austerity as preached by Buddha.

In the palpable absence of material possession and comfort, I could engage with the world around me intimately. I felt the snow on my fingers, the crisp mountain wind against my skin, and I realized how little we actually need to survive, and moreover, to be content.

Every step downwards was a lesson in humility, every stumble a reminder of the impermanence of our victories. The Buddhist philosophy of non-attachment illuminates how our attachments to the material world and our accomplishments can foster discontentment. The mountain taught me that by surrendering these emotional baggage, we can find true peace even in adversity.

11.3. Mindfulness Amidst Nature

Buddhism is deeply intertwined with nature, and the act of climbing and descending is, needless to say, an immersive experience in the wilderness. This allowed me to practice mindfulness, watch my every step, listen to my every breath, indulge in every bite of my sparse high-altitude meal, and feel the earth beneath me as I descended.

In the mind-numbing silence and physical exhaustion, I found the perfect sanctuary to put Buddha's principle of mindfulness into practice. Every breath was an opportunity to be aware of existence - of myself, the rugged landscape that I was so privileged to tread, the cosmic balance that allowed a delicate piece of life such as myself to survive in such an inhospitable environment.

11.4. The Essence of Impermanence

Buddha's teachings of impermanence reference the fleeting nature of existence that often escapes our immediate understanding. While climbing, it's easy to assume that the mountains have been there forever and always would be. The descent, however, revealed how even the mighty mountains are not immune from the passage of time - a landslide here, an eroded cliff there, and glaciers melting away more rapidly than ever.

Embracing impermanence allows us to appreciate each moment and each experience for its individual beauty, for its uniqueness, and for its ephemeral existence. Nothing remains stationary, and this brings the mind closer to the concept of cessation of suffering, or 'Nirvana.'

11.5. The Human Odyssey

Descending from the lofty peaks, I realized that the journey of mountaineering echoed the journey of life in equal measures. We ascend, we reach the zenith, and then we descend, mirroring the cycle of life and death. In between, we experience all the joys and sorrows, triumphs and betrayals, gain and loss, hand in hand.

Descending was indeed a physical manifestation of the Buddhist doctrine of the Middle Path, the balance between self-denial and self-indulgence. It was a demonstration that victory is only half the journey. The other, often overlooked half, lay in gracious acceptance of the descent, the return to reality, fashioned with the wisdom and strength gained from our victories.

Every ending is a new beginning, and so it was with the descent from the mountains. It marks the end of a climbing journey and a cascade into a whole new dimension of spiritual and personal enlightenment. As the saying goes, when one peak is scaled, another beckons. The journey is endless, as is the pursuit of enlightenment.

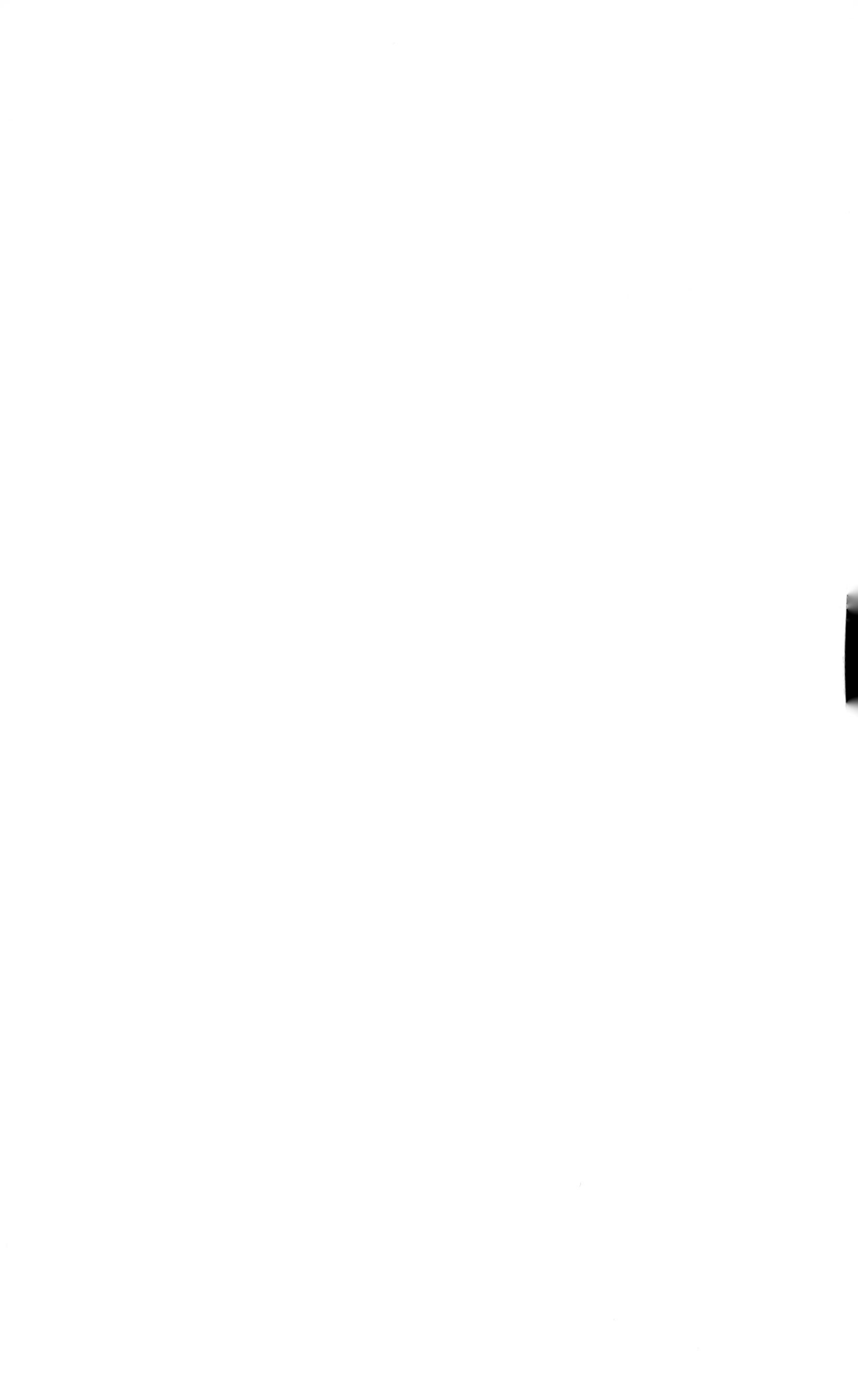